Healing By Faith

Keniysha J. Watts

ZYIA CONSULTING
Illuminate & Transcend

Dedication

This book is dedicated to all of my warrior sisters who have survived, lost, or in the fight against cancer and strived to rise above this ugly disease through faith and strength. May God strengthen your mind, body and spirit.

Acknowledgment

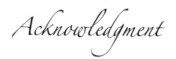

This book would not have been brought to light if it were not for God's divine journey that He placed me upon. To have blessed me with an amazing husband of seven years along with friendship of fourteen, Kenneth Watts, Jr. I couldn't have asked God for such an amazing partner to go through life with, and to take care of me through sickness and death, for richer or poor. You were created solely for me, and I cherish every moment I have with you. You stole my heart at the tender age of fifteen. We have been riding side by side since, no matter what tried to tear us apart. You never left my side, and I am forever grateful for your undying love. Now, here we are on the other side, winning together, and taking over like we always dreamed of. It will always be us, Bonnie & Clyde.

To my world, Keiden, Serenity, and Zacchaeus, mommy loves you dearly. I thank you all for allowing me to be your mother and best friend. Together we overcame what was sent to take us out. But, we are unstoppable with the strength we have together. As you all continue to grow and set out for greatness, I am right by your sides every step of the way. We are #WattsSquad.

To my Grandfather, Alfred Merrill, I thank you for being such an amazing man for our entire family. You have shown me what a real man is made of, and how to never sweat the small things in life, but to live with no fear, and love and trust God every step of the way. You will always be my messy granddaddy, and I will always be your Secretary.

To my Aunt Nese Grooms, I will forever treasure our bond and the love you pour out for not only me, but for my family as well. You've prayed for me and with me, when I couldn't find the strength to do for myself, all while giving me that space to embrace the journey God set me upon to grow into the woman God created me to be.

To my girls, Roberta (Berta), Kristen, Aisha, and Dejane, I thank you for being my rock when I needed it the most. You girls have gotten me through some of the darkest days with your encouraging words, prayers, visits and calls. I cannot thank you all enough. When I hit that mill, just know y'all getting a piece. Forever my sister's circle.

Table of Content

Healing By Faith

Introduction

December 31, 2019, was the day that changed my life forever. This day placed me on a journey so ugly, but so beautiful, that only God could have prepared me for such a graceful ending. I didn't know I would be faced with such a challenging task of shame, anger, bitterness and unconditional love. That sunny afternoon, as I left my in-law's home with my husband and three babies heading home to Atlanta, Georgia, we received the call from the hospital; I, Keniysha J. Watts, had stage three breast cancer at the age of twenty-eight years old. As the nurse on the other end talked to me, I was listening, but somewhere else at that moment. I was so shocked at how calm she gave me the news; no sympathy.

Nurse: Hi, this is Monica from Emory. Is this Keniysha?

Me: Yes, it is.

Nurse: Well we have your results, it shows you have Breast Cancer.

Me: Ok, I do.

Nurse: Yes, and we will have another nurse call you to set up your next appointment to see the oncologist. Thank you. Have a good day.

That was how the last day of 2019 ended. It changed my life forever. I was not mad or sad. Honestly, I didn't know how I felt. I just looked over at my husband and said, "Well, what a way to end our year and bring in the new year." I had just lost my grandmother less than a year to cancer, and had a baby seven months prior. From that moment on, I had tunnel vision with the news I had just received. I knew it was for a greater purpose that I would find out about along the journey.

As I looked over at my husband, I told him to take me to my grandparents' house to give the news to my family that they all had been waiting on as well. As we pulled into the yard, I felt like I was floating. Not really there, but there. If that makes sense. My grandfather and aunt were in the family room, sitting around waiting for my big news. Once I told them the news about my cancer diagnosis, it was like a blow to the stomach.

As I said earlier, my grandmother, Barbara Merrill, passed away in January 2019 from cancer. Now, here I am, the eldest grandchild, being diagnosed with cancer not even a year later. The journey we took with her was a rocky one.

She was the matriarch of the family; our rock. She was the woman who held our entire family together.

As I saw the look on my grandfather's face, it crushed me. But, I knew I had to be strong not only for him, but also for myself. I knew God was placing us on this oh-so-familiar journey, yet again. But this time, we were more equipped. We now had a strong guardian angel to guide us through.

As I take you through this healing journey, I will also unravel how my faith was tested and ultimately saved me from this ugly disease called cancer.

Chapter One
20/20 Vision

We all have our goals and dreams mapped out as the new year approaches. We set out for it to be better than the previous year. We are more intentional, strive for success in different ways, whether financially, in our marriages, or in friendships. Then you have me, who wrote down goals and dreams for the new year to start new businesses, revamp existing ones, and overall start off on a new journey in Atlanta, Georgia. But instead, here I was laying in my husband's arms, sobbing because I had just gotten the worst news of my life.

How could this be? I'm only twenty-eight years old, and have three small children to take care of. Will I be able to survive this? Man, my grandma just passed away not even a year ago. There were so many thoughts that came into my mind as I lay there. My vision of what I had set out to achieve seemed so cloudy. But, just as I was about to think even more depressing thoughts, God spoke to me and said, "This is not unto death my child. You will live and not die." I heard God speak to me clear as day. And, it changed my entire outlook on the whole situation. See, I have always been a strong-minded person. Even as a little girl, I never let devastating situations get the best of me.

Just to give you a little background of my life, I am the oldest and first grandchild on my mother and father's side of the family. I am also the daughter of two amazing parents who birthed me at the young age of seventeen years old. I was very loved and protected throughout my childhood. However, at the age of eight, I became a victim of domestic violence and molestation by a man I called daddy. He was not my biological father. He was my step-father whom my mother was married to at the time.

For seven years, she also was a victim of his domestic abuse. My mother and I went through a great deal of violence. It hurt me so much that I was unable to help her. I became very afraid of letting anyone know what was happening. I never could understand why my mother stayed so long and endured so much pain and suffering. But, it was not my battle to fight, nor understand at such a young age.

Many nights, I would hide in my closet to escape the abuse that was happening to my mother, hoping and praying that I would not be next in line. How could a man that is supposed to be your protector be the complete opposite and have no remorse for his actions? That was something I could never quite grasp, and it bothered me for years to come. Having to keep so much bottled in, afraid to talk with anyone about what had happened to me over the years became very challenging. I was no longer afraid to speak my truth, even if it would turn out good or bad, or if anyone would believe me.

Several times, I would try and muster up the courage to tell my mom, but I always would be too afraid to tell her. I couldn't shake the fact that she had been in the same situation as me. So, how would she be able to help me when she was unable to help herself. Even though he had been sent to prison for abusing my mother, to the point she almost lost her life, I was still so angry at the fact that nothing had been done about what had been done to me. Nevertheless, I had to find the courage and speak up.

For many years, I kept quiet about the situation. I never told my mother or father, until I was sixteen years old. I was unable to keep such a heavy burden any longer. Up until that time, I never blamed anyone for what happened to me, nor did I shame myself for it. I knew the situation did not define me, and would not detour the purpose God had for me.

Once I told my parents what had taken place, I was a bit taken back by the responses I received. At that moment, I regretted saying anything and immediately went into a shell. What I expected from my parents was an overwhelming urge to seek justice. Instead, it was a response of shock and unbelief. From that day on, neither my parents nor I talked about the situation, or how it had affected me over the years. The situation was a lot to take in. I was not going to continue to dwell in the past, but I would thrive through it.

My past was now my past. And, no matter what I had been through, nothing was going to keep me down or consume me with the dark areas of my life. I also understood that I was not the only one to have been through such a traumatizing past. So many others came through many obstacles and soared despite all that had been against them.

My parents loved me, and wanted nothing but the best for me. Unfortunately, they were not able to protect me from the evil and danger that was right in our home. As strong as I was, I coached myself daily to have a strong mindset no matter the diagnosis or what the doctors would say. I had such a strong will to overcome this so-called death sentence that so many around me claimed it to be.

Many times, people would tell me how bad cancer is amongst women, and that I was going to die if I didn't do what the doctors told me to do. I would also hear that I couldn't heal my cancer on my own. I would constantly hear how I needed the doctor to help me beat cancer, and the food and herbal supplements wouldn't be enough. Those who spoke these words were people who didn't take the best care of themselves and solely depended on the doctors for everything.

I had to have a real heart-to-heart conversation with God as to how he wanted me to go about my healing. These words constantly ran through my mind, "Healing By Faith."

God healed me, not man. I no longer had the vision of what I had planned to do for the year. My focus was on the vision God had planned out for me that I had no insight into how it would go. I was no longer in control of what was happening in my life. I had to adjust to a new chapter.

It all seemed so familiar, but I had a sense of calmness that I had such a great person on my side to guide and care for me throughout the journey. I knew God had a special assignment for me. I was determined to find out what it would come to be. No matter what I knew, I was chosen for a purpose that was bigger than me. It was no coincidence that I had been diagnosed with cancer, not even a year after laying my grandmother to rest. I knew that I would be up against a battle. Nevertheless, I would not have to fight alone.

Knowing this gave me comfort and peace. I had The Creator on my side. I couldn't allow the diagnosis to overcome me to the point that I would be so consumed with the fear of not living. That mindset would definitely take me out of here, and that was not going to happen. Self-control was possible, if I allowed myself to think on positive notions and not negative ones. Still, I was unsure of what to do, or what I was up against. But, God had me under his loving arms to protect me from the fears I had running through my mind.

The Choice

As we all know, 20/20 vision is clear and unfiltered. I was going into the new year of 2020 with a vision that I had not put together. However, it was the one God wanted for me. I had no choice but to see it through without clarity of where it would lead me. That's where the faith kicked in to allow God to lead me every step of the way throughout my journey of cancer.

I had never heard of anyone seeing God in the flesh, and nor had I. I have heard many stories of how God showed up in some of the most bizarre situations when they least expected God to show up. My relationship with God became very personal. It was a bond that I had to allow myself to accept without all the notions and opinions of others. God's vision for me was not for anyone else to understand; why I would make the decisions I would make or lose some very special people along the way.

My vision of the life I always dreamed of having wasn't impossible. Now, I was on a path that I did not choose for myself. However, it was the path I knew was necessary for where God was taking me.

Have you ever sat down and wrote all your dreams and goals, maybe weekly, monthly or yearly? But, in the midst of you marking them off, one by one, there's a detour due to something out of your control. Well, that was me. I wasn't ready for half of the things I was about to embark on.

I had no clue what I was facing. But, I trusted God with everything in me. I had to trust myself that I would and could get through everything that was about to happen, whether I liked it or not. I had to focus on God's grace for me to overcome this season of my life. It wasn't a shout of a doubt that I wouldn't accomplish this new set goal that I had not planned or set out to do. God gave me such a goal he knew I was built to accomplish it, no matter how bad things would look or feel.

Now, here I was adding this to my goal list "Total Healing" in my mind and heart. I look at the journey being a breeze and no harm done to me. I believed in my heart that the cancer would not leave the area it originally formed in, and if I decided to take chemotherapy it would do what it needed to be done while not making me sick. I prayed to God day in and day out that my requests would be met. I had things to do and this was not my plan. Like a woman says, God said, "I got this. I got this, just follow my lead. Don't worry. You will be rewarded if you keep me first and trust me all the way through."

Oftentimes, I couldn't help but to get in my mind and question everything about this situation. It was like, how can I be going through this right now at this moment. I had seen what cancer had done to my Grandma less than a year prior, and I hated it with a passion. Cancer is a beast, and it has no remorse for nothing or nobody.

During these times, I asked God, "Why me? How could

you put me in the same position that took my Grandmother away? How could this build me up and not tear me down? Where would this leave me after it's all over? Will I be able to be myself again?"

Yes, I had many questions for my Creator. I knew he could give me the answers. I mean, he was the one who orchestrated the entire journey from beginning to end. I had choices either to trust him and think positive thoughts about the journey, or be mad, scared and desperate. I had some decisions to make and they weren't that easy to pick. I wanted to be all of them in one. I wanted to trust God with all my heart, but I was angry and scared of the unknown. And, that was something I hated so badly.

Here I was, on my knees praying, and pleading with God about all of my wants and needs. I demanded him to fulfill them for my life. I believed my life depended on it. I knew I needed him to get me through it all. I had faith in myself, but it wasn't as strong as it should have been and that scared me. I knew, as a child, I could always count on myself if everything else failed. I was the only person who could truly hold me back from accomplishing anything in my life. But, here I was, not so sure if I could honestly have that same strong faith that I have always had to believe I would be just fine going into this journey I wasn't ready for.

I Can

Having faith in something you have never seen can be a bit uneasy. But, knowing the one who created you, let's you know it can only turn out to be a blessing in the end. The vision I had thought I wanted for myself was no longer there. I was okay with that, because 2020 would be a year to remember forever. I pulled myself together to be strong for myself and my family. I couldn't allow a disease to take me out of here. Especially, without leaving an imprint on my babies.

They were young; three, five and seven months old. That was way too young for them to easily forget their mother. The vision became clear to me; no matter what, I will fight and fight hard and be here for my family. They needed to see that mommy was going to become their superwoman. Most of all, they just didn't know they were becoming the biggest part of my journey.

My children became the fuel to my fire to push me through this unforeseen season of our lives. They were very young, but also very aware of things starting to change all around us. They saw how mommy was at her peak of good health then became tired quickly; from being able to run around and chase them for hours without being tired, cooking without becoming lightheaded and having to sit while cooking, to being tired in short periods of time. At times, they began asking, "Mommy are you ok?" I would always reply, "Yes, mommy is just a little tired. There is nothing to worry about."

I do believe kids can sense things sometimes before we adults do. I know for me, I trust my kids' intuitions; my baby boy, Zaccheaus, was the one who made me aware of my lump in my breast.

At six months, he abruptly stopped nursing. We were so attached, during the time I had been nursing him. It was such a special bond to hold my baby boy and be able to nurture him from the body I had also carried him in. I immediately sensed something was off when he stopped nursing. Especially, when our nursing sessions were always good.

One evening, I stood in the shower, felt my breast, and noticed a hard and large knot. My mind went to just a few years prior after I had my daughter, Serenity. I was able to breastfeed her for five months until my milk supply stopped. I had also felt a small knot in my breast then. I had it checked out through an ultrasound and was told it was benign. They told me it was a clogged milk duct and nothing to worry about since I had just stopped breastfeeding and was only 25 years old.

I was too young for a mammogram. So, this go around I didn't think much of it since I had been through the same situation as before. I looked up several different remedies to release the potential clogged milk duct. But as time went by, weeks turned into months and nothing was helping;

only me experiencing pain and discomfort. I can't say to you that I wasn't worried, because I was. I was very much attuned with my body. I could always find the littlest things that maybe off or not in order with what I've always known it to be.

In November of 2019, I drove five hours, alone, to a childhood friend's funeral in my hometown of Pensacola, Florida. I was in deep thought the entire time, wondering if the knot in my breast could be something more than just a knot. I had never experienced pain in my breast besides having engorged breasts from needing to pump milk out to feed my children. That night, as I drove down the interstate, it was a pain and feeling I couldn't shake. I had already called into the breast center to have myself checked, once I got back home to Atlanta to rule out anything alarming.

As I visited my hometown, no one knew how much pain I was in. I smiled, laughed and celebrated his life with other friends I had grown up with. I would go off to the restroom to let out a scream that I kept in while around everyone, just to come back to the crowd like nothing had been wrong. Once the funeral was over, I eventually told two of my friends that I had been experiencing pain, and I had an appointment setup once I returned home. They both reminded me to let them know the results once I received them.

When I returned home to my family, it was like a whirl-wind effect. It seemed like no matter what I tried to do to relieve the pain nothing seemed to work. My first appointment was uncomfortable, but similar to the appointment I had a few years prior. I received the same diagnosis that it was a possible clogged milk duct. But, this appointment ended differently, and it made me think more into it.

The doctor prescribed me antibiotics to clear out a possible breast infection. I was prescribed to take them for seven days. By day five, I couldn't take the pain any longer and the antibiotics were making me sick. I called to book another appointment to see what could be the problem. I was scheduled to come in the day before Christmas Eve, December 23, 2019. Instead of me preparing for my family's first Christmas in our new home, I was heading to have a biopsy done, and didn't expect to go through the worst day of my life.

My husband, right by my side and holding my hand, I felt confident that whatever was going on in my body was being taken care of that day. The nurse called me to come to the back, without my husband, only me. I walked into a slightly dimmed room with a semi-surgical table to lay on. The nurse introduced herself and assured me I would be just fine, and there would be nothing to worry about.

As the doctor came in and introduced herself, I asked questions as to what was to be expected from the biopsy. She stated to me that there were some concern about my breast and the biopsy would detect from the tissue taken if it would be anything alarming. I layed there with the nurse alking to me through the procedure. I heard a few clicks, out no pain until I felt a stab so sharp I almost jumped off the table.

The doctor had hit my muscle, and it was very painful. She immediately apologized and tried to calm me down. I could tell she may have been alarmed as well from how I responded. The procedure ended, which felt like it took forever. I walked into the waiting room to my husband. We drove home to be with our babies, and continue to prepare for Christmas in the days to come.

By Christmas day, I was in excruciating pain. I barely could get around, was very fatigued, and sore all over my body. I was able to prepare our Christmas dinner with the help of my husband and grandmother who had come to spend the holidays with us. Our first Christmas was a very special day for us and we enjoyed every bit of it.

The next day, we got on the road to spend a few days with family in our hometown, with every intention not to worry ourselves about anything concerning my previous doctor's appointments. Our trip back to our hometown was beautiful. We celebrated the life of my late grandmother, Barbara, who had recently passed earlier in the year.

A few of my family members were aware I had been experiencing breast pain, but weren't concerned, just as I was not. But, to our avail, the last day of the year, we all were hit with unexpected news that no one was prepared for. I can vividly remember the entire events leading up to that day and it just shows how much our lives can be turned upside down within a blink of an eye.

When we get devastating news, we don't seem to see things clearly. We question our entire life, inch by inch. I felt deep down in my soul that being diagnosed with cancer would forever change my life. I wasn't worried, because I knew God was with me, and I'd be ok. So, yes, going into the new year of 2020, the vision I had for myself wasn't exactly what God had planned. However, I knew he had something bigger in store for me.

Chapter Two
The Unknown

On January 13, 2020, my husband and I were told that I had stage three breast cancer. To hear what stage and the actual name of the cancer were shocking. The oncologist told us that it was Invasive Mammary Carcinoma Stage 3. In a nutshell, it is an aggressive cancer that could possibly take my life, if I didn't follow their lead. Most doctors will tell you if you don't start a treatment plan right away and follow their recommendations, then the cancer will only progress and you will eventually die from it.

I had been through this journey as a caretaker, but not as a patient. Now, here I was as a patient unfamiliar with the different terms and angles that were being brought forth to me. My husband sat next to me taking it all in quietly, as always. I could see that he wasn't bothered by the conversation the doctor was having with us. We weren't afraid of the diagnosis and we definitely weren't taking the doctor's word as law.

What I did not know beforehand was how forceful the doctors were going to be to make me choose a decision so quickly. I felt like I was on the hot seat to make such a life-changing decision in such a short time. I needed to have the time to process everything I had been presented with over the course of only a few days. Why would I agree to something so drastic and not be given a chance to research or even give me the space to ask probing questions about the treatment plan that would be created for me to possibly beat cancer with? I didn't know what exactly the treatment would be doing to my body.

The doctor just went on and on about how I have to act fast and be aggressive with such aggressive cancer that has attacked my body. There was no sympathy in the conversation, only that "Hey, you're young. You will bounce back quicker than most women." I'm looking this man straight in his face like what kind of person says that like it's an ok thing to say to someone.

I couldn't help but wonder how many other women have sat where I was sitting and felt like another number to this same man. Did they also feel just like another patient who was just passing through? I asked myself, does this man even care about what I want? He sure hasn't asked me from the time he has come into this office until now.

So many thoughts were running through my mind. Honestly, I had kind of checked out of the majority of his conversation. See, I'm a strong-willed woman who you can't just tell me to do something without giving me the opportunity to ask questions and to also know who you are as a person. Especially, with you being so up close and personal with me for a long period of time in my life. Cancer treatment isn't a one day, one week, or even a one month ordeal. It takes weeks, months, and sometimes years of dealing with doctors and other healthcare workers.

I am big on building solid trustworthy relationships with people who would be having a big impact on my body and my life decisions. I had seen many relatives fall victim to giving complete power over to a doctor, just because of the title they hold. Many of them were too scared to ask questions or not ask enough questions pertaining to their health. I had seen many people, in my family and my community, fall victim to their doctor's orders. I vowed to never allow them to have such an impact on me as it had upon them. It's a saying, "When you know better, you do better." I knew I wasn't going to allow a doctor to just give me what they wanted to give me without a complete explanation on how their curated treatment plan would be in my best interest.

This doctor clearly didn't care as to what I thought. He was just there to do his job; tell me how he was going to give me a chance to live longer, how he planned to do so with a treatment plan that had been around for many years, but has been far more effective in the last fifteen to twenty years. I can't say I agreed with everything he was saying. I had still seen many women die from the same treatment plan he so desperately wanted me to start on right away.

It made me angry that he and so many other doctors showed no empathy or sympathy for their patients as they should. How could you be in such a position over someone's life and not have an ounce of kindness to someone who is going through such a life-changing moment, and at such a young age? And, to think of all the many women who were in these appointments by themselves with no support whatsoever. To only have a man in a white coat sell you a "second chance at life," but it comes with so many other life-altering complications and so-called second chance that you don't understand how you even got to this place in the first place. I know if I was thinking these thoughts, I know so many other women had thought the same thoughts as me.

The doctor was so shocked that I didn't shed a tear. Instead, I uttered the words. ''God has the last say," with a smile on my face. He then went on to say, ''You want to be here for your babies, and do all that you can to be here for them.'' Yes, I did without a shadow of a doubt. My kids are my everything. As I looked at them, playing around in the doctor's office, and I knew I couldn't leave them. And, I wasn't.

The question the doctor asked was so vague. It made me feel some type of way. Like, how dare you ask me a no-brainer question like that. Who wouldn't want to be here for their children? I nor anyone else asked to be diagnosed with a deadly disease that has the whole world shook at just the sound of it. Many types of research have been done on the various types of cancers and millions, if not billions, of dollars, have been raised and distributed to many organizations to find a cure for this ugly disease. Yet, still no cure or not even a solid answer as to how or why a person has cancer.

So many theories and so many are left in the unknown of not knowing how the cancer started. Was it the food? Was it hereditary, stress-related, or some sort of trauma that triggered it to manifest? I, myself, had so many questions. However, I knew this particular doctor wasn't the one to give me the answers I was seeking. His delivery wasn't about how to heal the body from the dis-ease, but more so to get rid of what was there and to potentially cut out whatever would be leftover.

My mind was going a million miles per sec at this very moment, thinking of my grandmother who had never smoked a day in her life, but was still diagnosed with stage four lung cancer. She was not aware that she had been living with cancer in her body for quite some time. I wondered how she felt after being diagnosed with advanced stage cancer. The doctors could not give her a straight answer as to how the cancer came about, only to start their treatment plan as soon as possible so she could live longer, only to have lost the battle two years later.

I know every person's diagnosis is different. However, having a system so dedicated to pushing such a powerful drug onto you so that you can live longer and not even guaranteed that you will is pretty messed up. I had watched my beautiful vibrant grandmother go from a strong courageous woman to somewhat helpless in such a short amount of time from the harsh treatment plan given. I didn't understand a lot of the terms that were given, but I was eager to learn for my understanding.

I wanted a doctor to not just tell me all the different terms, but to also educate me on what they were. I asked the doctor a few questions in regards to the cancer stage as to how long I had the cancer. He responded that it could have possibly been there for years, seeing how large the tumor was. My take on it was it couldn't have been so with me just finding the lump in my breast just within the last two months of the diagnosis. I had breastfed my baby boy for four months with no prior issues. I wanted answers.

I was not getting the answers I wanted, and it upset me very much. I was always under the notion that you go to the doctors when there is something wrong, and you are needing assistance in what can alleviate the problem. The doctor isn't the one to heal the body, but one to give guidance into the healing process. See, the doctor has his job to analyze and assist me in beating the cancer, but they also always say the treatments aren't guaranteed. I would have to always follow up on my progress yearly. I knew what God had told me and that was, "It isn't unto death."

The doctor threw around all the terms for how aggressive the cancer was and said what all he was going to do. Not once did he ask me how I felt or what steps I wanted to take. Once again, here I was being told by a total stranger, who I had just met that I would have to go through sixteen rounds of chemotherapy, a mastectomy, radiation, and at the end of it all, I would still need to take a chemotherapy pill for at least five years. Not to mention, I would be able to have a "nice boob job" (his words). All of which was just the initial step into treating the cancer that may still be there after going through this intense treatment plan recommended.

After about forty-five minutes into the appointment, I had made the decision I didn't want him as my doctor. I did not feel good about his presence. So, I told him I'd be in touch once my husband and I talked over everything. I left the doctor's office feeling numb. I didn't know what to do or where to begin. I was twenty-seven years old, never had been sick a day in my life, nor ever hospitalized besides from having kids. Yet, here I was faced with so many decisions to make and unsure which route to take.

I can honestly say I was very uncomfortable with doctors, especially white doctors. The majority of doctors in my city were white old men and women who had been around for decades and were racist and it showed. I had always been seen by a white doctor growing up and very seldom seen a doctor of my color or culture. Many of my encounters were not too pretty. I had been dismissed when explaining the issues and concerns I was having, or even the pain I had been enduring to only be advised to take a Tylenol in which I needed medical attention instead.

Here I am, a young black woman, talking to this older white man, who may have a history of racism in his family. He may not care less about my well-being, but is working to get a check and send me on my way. There was nothing we could relate to. And, that was a big part of me searching for a doctor to feel comfortable and appreciated, so I would not feel that I was just another black girl with cancer.

I told myself that I would be just fine, and find the right doctor to guide me through everything. I just needed to hear from God. I shut myself away from family and friends. My husband and I went into an intensive prayer and fasted for twenty-one days. During that time, I was going back and forth to doctor's appointments from second opinions to plastic surgeons and also holistic/alternative doctors. I had changed my diet drastically, going cold turkey on consuming sugars, meats, alcohol and dairy. In which I had learned was one of many key factors of healing from cancer. It was a difficult thing to do, but I was determined to try whatever it was to overcome the cancer. Also from my understanding of the Bible fasting and praying, it is a very sacred step into healing from sickness and disease within the mind and body.

Every day, I was constantly searching for information on how to beat cancer, what are the causes of cancer, nutrition for cancer and so much more. I was allowing the cancer to consume me, which was not a good thing. I couldn't shake the fact that I had been diagnosed with breast cancer, and didn't understand where it had come from. From my research, I found that processed food could cause cancer along with everyday household products I had been using my entire life. So, instead of me focusing on what may have caused it, I decided to focus my time and energy on being at peace and working towards healing my body, as much as I could.

I dedicated time to talk with God so I could hear him give me the right steps to take. See, I come from an amazing family who believes in the power of prayer and seeking God's guidance in every aspect of life. My personal relationship with God is like me talking to my best friend, but a best friend who created me and knows me better than I know myself and one I can trust.

After our 21-day fast, I got the clarity and confirmation I needed; not to do chemotherapy. Making that decision was a battle. My grandmother had passed away from cancer just a year prior to my diagnosis. And, I saw how she had taken all the treatments from start to finish and was told she was in remission being that the cancer was gone. But, then it returned to another part of her body and the doctor saying nothing can be done was so devastating to my family and grandmother. My family and I tried to incorporate some holistic approaches to help aid in her healing, but in order for it to work properly, that individual has to want to do it and has to have self-discipline and be consistent.

I had told myself, during the time she was dealing with cancer, that if I ever had cancer I would go on a holistic approach to getting rid of the cancer. So, when God spoke to me and said no chemotherapy, I was happy. I was afraid of the treatment and did not want to go through what my grandmother had gone through. I didn't know what God had planned for me, during this journey, but I trusted him without knowing what was ahead of me.

Not knowing was a pet peeve of mine. I always wanted to be in control and know every detail. However, cancer has a mind of its own, and it can kill you if you allow it. I wasn't about to let that happen. I put all my faith in God and buckled my seat for the ride of my life not knowing how long and where this journey would take me.

Chapter Three
Time

As time moved on, my faith was tested and it came with a price. I will forever keep it as a memory of what not to do. After I received the word from God, not to do chemotherapy, I enlightened my close family and friends about my decision. Some were on board with my decision and others were not. The ones who did not agree had no problem telling me that I had made a bad choice. I was told that I should listen to the doctors, because they were right. And, I shouldn't take my life into my own hands, but allow the doctors to do what they needed to do. Whatever that meant.

I continued to hear this over and over again to the point I became scared. I became afraid to go without chemotherapy, even though I knew what God had told me. I allowed the negative conversations to pierce, break me down, and give in.

My husband was so disappointed in me, because God had given him the same word. He wanted me to step back, lean and depend on God. All of this happened only a couple of weeks after our 21-day fast. I couldn't see that the enemy was attacking my mind through some of my closest loved ones.

On February 20, 2020, I went in to have my port put in my upper right chest area. It would be connected to a large vein that the chemotherapy would be administered through. I had a friend, at the time, take me to get the procedure done. I was nervous, but not scared. As I was being prepped to go into surgery, my nurse asked me if I had tried or looked into any other options besides chemo. My response was yes. But, honestly, I became frightened at the unknown of whether it would cure me or not.

I explained to her how I had changed my diet and allowed God to guide me in my steps through healing the cancer. I confessed to her that God told me not to take chemo as a treatment. Nevertheless, I was going against his instructions, because I allowed family and friends to drive fear into me. She looked at me and said, 'If you know what God has told you not to do, then why are you here? Why are you being disobedient?" The only answer I could give her was that I was scared and didn't want to die.

I had become so comfortable in my fear that even through this complete stranger God was still trying to guide me. I was being disobedient to God's instructions out of fear. After our talk, they wheeled me to the operating room to place my port in for my first chemo treatment following the next week.

On February 27, 2020, I went into the cancer center with

a positive attitude. I actually was pleased with my doctor. The fact that he was black really put my mind at ease. As I sat there with my husband, he asked me if this was something I really wanted to do. I said to him I have to do what I have to do to live and that was that. I walked into the room with other patients receiving infusions. All of them were older and nowhere in sight was a person my age. I sat there for five hours having this poison invade my body in hopes of killing the cancer cells.

As I looked over at my husband, I felt happy that he was by my side. So, many others were there alone with no support. As I awakened, after a few hours of being knocked out from all the medications, I slowly came to. I was released for the day, to return in a few days for my checkup. I stood up and instantly became ill. I told my nurse I wasn't feeling too good. They assured me it was likely from all the medications, and once I ate a little something and rested I would be fine.

My husband and I stopped and ate lunch, then headed to pick up our son from school. I felt like I was going to puke all over the place. And, that was exactly what I did as soon as we arrived home. For six days straight I vomited, unable to eat or drink anything. I couldn't get out of the bed without my husband carrying me to and from the bathroom. On the second day of being home from my first round of chemo, I received a phone call from a private number. I was unable to answer the call due to how weak I was. The person left a voicemail. It was my doctor checking on me to see how things were going. I found it kind of odd that he would be calling at such a time outside of office hours and also calling so discreetly.

On day three, I was rushed to the ER to have emergency fluids. My five-year-old son and husband sat with me for hours that night, in a small chair trying to get some sleep. I could barely talk, because of how weak I was. I saw the sadness in my baby's face, seeing his mom so sick and weak. I had been pumped with liters upon liters of saline fluids to hydrate me. I was extremely dehydrated from not being able to drink any water due to my excessive vomiting. After hours of being there, I was released late in the night to return home.

By day four, I had not gained any strength and was unable to hold anything down, constantly vomiting. I called my doctor. They advised me to go into a nearby infusion center to receive fluids again. My husband was away at school, an hour away from home. With no family to call, I called a church member to take me and she came right away. She stayed with me until I was checked in, and came back once I finished. I was hoping that the fluids would help me, but they did not.

That night, as I lay in bed, I had a dream so clear that I thought I was dead. In my dream, I stood in my grandmother's kitchen, which was her sanctuary. A place where she not only cooked for our family, but was also her outlet when she needed to let off some steam. I saw her at her kitchen sink. She did not acknowledge me. I asked her what was wrong and she told me she was upset with me, because I wasn't supposed to take the chemotherapy treatment. I knew she was right. I was so ashamed. Here I was fighting for my life, because I decided to allow people to get into my ear and deter me from what I knew I was not supposed to do. I had lost my faith, because of fear of the unknown.

By day five, I didn't know if I was dying or living. This particular day, I lay in bed, unable to open my eyes. I went into a daze where I found myself at my grandmother's funeral. I walked in, sat down, and just stared at the casket. I felt someone sit beside me dressed in all white. As I looked to the left of me, I saw the face of my grandmother. She smiled and held me. She told me she was with me, and that I would be just fine. She also told me that God was disappointed in me, but he is still with me, and would continue to guide me through my journey.

I felt my body rise from the bed. When I opened my eyes, I saw my husband and son standing beside me. They sat there with me and I explained what I had experienced. From that moment, I knew I was not alone and going to be just fine.

By day six, I was able to gain strength and walk outside. I told my husband I would not continue chemo. See, I was so stuck on the what if's and the negative talks that I didn't give God the time to do what needed to be done. I mean,

I began with faith in God, but soon as I hit a dark spot, I doubted what he could do. In making that decision out of fear, I almost lost my life not giving God the time that was needed.

Chapter Four
Healing By Faith

Can we say I had a wake-up call? When God tells you not to do something, I suggest you listen and do as he says. I will not say I always listen to what God tells me to do or don't do without thinking twice. Even though I know deep down God will make a way and protect me. But, it is something trying to allow a higher being take control, and you are at ease with it.

I can take you back to my childhood. When I would go to church with my grandmother, she would preach and lay hands on others. Many came to her for strength or even healing. I had the notion that it was a miracle when she and others would pray and lay hands on the sick. They would come back to church giving their testimony of how God had used them to heal their bodies.

I did not know, at the time, what it really meant to have faith. It took me to go through my very own journey of healing to learn about having faith. I had to learn how to step out of the way to allow God to take control and trust him. Him being the creator, he knows what's best.

My faith had been rocked. I had not been doing everything in my power to stay positive. It took me a few weeks to regroup, but I was back into my Bible, and seeking guidance from God. I no longer allowed anyone to speak fear into me. However, faith without work is dead, right? I was being consistent with my nutrition, exercise, and kept negative people and things out of my life. I had to find the strength to be strong for my kids and allow myself to have total healing.

As I sat in my home, in Atlanta, Georgia, I thought about how we were without our family. I had a few close friends who were of great help, but had their own families to take care of. Here I was home, alone, with our oldest son who was only five years old. During this time, my husband attended school an hour away from us, five days a week.

I had to find the strength and create a game plan to take care of myself and bring our two youngest children back home from Florida. They were missing their mom and ready to come home. I was ready to have my babies back with me as well. Also, my five-year-old son was scared to death of what he had witnessed after his mommy had taken chemo.

With everything that was going on, I had so many emotions. Amongst those emotions was anger. I was angry because I did not have all of my kids with me. We had to send our youngest kids to Florida so I could start chemo. We did not have anyone to help take care of them. I was angry because I didn't ask for this and now I'm fighting for my life with the natural uncertainty of if I will beat it or will it take my life away. I was battling a disease and not sure what to do.

I was going back and forth in my mind. Once again, I hear a voice say, "Healing By Faith." I wrote it down, and told my husband about it. We both said that this would be a part of my journey; "Healing By Faith." I had to have crazy faith. The type of faith that no matter what the circumstances may look like, holding on to the word that God had given me and my family, would bring me to a place in my life to give my testimony on how God's grace and favor brought me through my challenging time.

I had already gone through my first battle, and wasn't sure if I would face anymore like it. My faith was that I would allow myself to ask and receive the guidance of God without worrying or contradicting myself if I made the right decision. I had to put in the work for it all to come together. I had to stay strong and stand on his word; he is the healer and provider for all my needs.

As I continued to lean and depend on God, things started to move in a way that I knew he was with me. My husband and I decided to shave my hair off, which was a very challenging thing to do. It was such a shock to me that from only having one treatment I had already started to lose my hair. When you are so used to having your hair your entire life and lose it, not by choice, it is heartbreaking.

So, as I sat in front of my husband and my son Keiden, I began to try and embrace the new journey of being bald and everything that came with it. I had faith that I would not look like this forever, and it would just be another chapter in my book of overcoming. Yet, another battle in life that didn't break me.

After my husband cut my hair, I opened my eyes for the first time. I looked in the mirror, at my reflection, in awe at this new look I was seeing in front of me. My son said, "Wow, mommy! You look like a warrior. You're beautiful." I was so amazed at how beautiful I was bald and realized my hair did not define me. I told myself I could embrace my natural beauty within and allow it to exude outward unapologetically.

Not many women have that confidence to accept such a drastic look when it's out of their control, and it weighs on them. Some of us do not feel beautiful without our hair on top of our heads. In so many cultures, the woman's crown is her hair. We are so proud to have hair and express ourselves through various types of styles and colors. But, some women like myself, accept the things that are out of our control and make the best out of the situation.

I could have instantly gone into a shell not wanting to live, looking at the worst possibility, with being diagnosed with cancer, trying to seek help and validation from every which way possible. But, why would I do that? Many people put all their trust into man when it comes to health, finances, and even our relationships. We've all fallen short of seeking help in one or more areas of our lives' troubles. However, when man falls short and is unable to help us or guide us, we then go running to God for help to fix the problem. We should always seek him first before anything else.

The scripture Hebrews 11:1 and 6 (ESV) says, "Now faith is assurance of things hoped for, the conviction of things not seen," / "And without faith it is impossible to please Him, for he who comes to God must believe that He is and that He is a rewarder of those who seek Him." That was what I strived to do; receive my reward for being faithful to obey God's word and guidance. I mean who wants to go through such an uncomfortable journey and receive nothing for being obedient.

My trust had to be solely in God and not myself. I could so easily get detoured from the right path that God has set forth for me. But, by following my own way, not knowing which path to go down could lead me to a more difficult path than I would like to take.

"Trust in the Lord with all your heart, and do not lean on your own understanding." ~ Proverbs 3:5-6

I can't lie to you and say I wasn't afraid of not knowing every detail that would transpire. Nevertheless, I knew the one and only person who knows me best, better than I knew myself; the one who created me through and through was amazing to me. So, I was determined to overcome every fear I had. I will be in great health and beat this ugly disease that has invaded my body. I Am Healed, I Am Beautiful, I am Blessed, I Am Anointed were the affirmations I spoke over myself daily.

I was determined to show up as my best self, care for my children, and not have any limitations doing so. As long as I keep a positive mind state I would be just fine. In doing so, I would need guidance on how to keep it going even when I may get discouraged at times.

I found my happy space with journaling my thoughts and prayers, meditating on God's word after I would read my Bible or daily devotions, listening to uplifting music, or even listening to music that made me get up and dance. I even found strength and peace when I would pray for others who would come to me for prayer. I felt honored that even total strangers would want me to pray for them in their times of need.

As my husband and I drove to Pensacola to pick up our children and bring them home for good, I prayed for God to give me a strength that I had never had before. No matter what, I would lean and depend on him through it all. It was an amazing feeling being back home in Atlanta; all of us together. I was now going to show my family and the world how "Healing By Faith" really looked flaws and all.

I was now back in my space, and going to take full

control over my life. I strived to get back to the basics of getting my mind, body, and spirit all the way together and not allow my emotions or the things I see to get me unfocused. I was my biggest competition, at this point. It was either allow the doctors to tell me what to do and how to do it or allow my creator, God, Jesus Christ, himself guide and lead me through it. And that's where my faith kicked into overdrive. All gas no breaks. It was time for me to get out of the way of myself and allow God to do his thing.

My faith and trust were knowing I would be just fine. Trusting God was the key to healing and thriving through the journey of cancer. I mean why not have confidence in someone or something other than a person or thing that doesn't know you, but will be there and show you an even better way of life.

Once I went back to my oncologist, I told him I would not continue any further chemotherapy. He didn't have much to say. He tried to explain that the type of aggressive cancer I had been diagnosed with could not be overcome without chemotherapy. I understood his position as a doctor. I also understood and knew, without a shadow of a doubt, that my God was even more aggressive. I politely thanked him, but wanted him to know and understand that God would have the last say so and not man.

My doctor wasn't letting up too easily by just letting me go. He assured me that he would try and lower my dosage so it would not affect me in such a harsh way like before. But, when I asked him how sure he was, he couldn't promise me that I wouldn't have the same side effects, but would work to try and limit the severity of them. As we went back and forth he politely said to me that if I didn't continue the treatments I would eventually be in bad shape and it could potentially be deadly for me. I declined his recommendations and he finally accepted my wishes. He wished me the best of luck and assured me that he would be available if I needed him.

As the days went by, I found various support groups through Facebook and Instagram. I made great connections with women in my community, who had or were overcoming breast cancer. It was amazing how well I bounced back from the chemo treatment that nearly took my life just a month earlier. I gained so much strength I felt as if nothing or no one could get me down with my crazy faith. I knew I was going to be just fine.

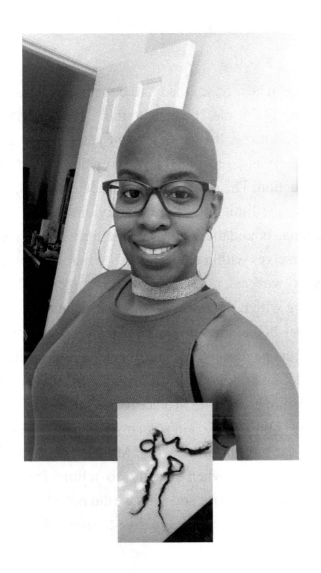

Chapter Five
Boundaries

When you hear or see the word boundaries, what comes to your mind? For me, it means to mind your business and don't come for me. If I haven't asked you for your help or opinion, there is no reason for you to place your thoughts on my situation. The real definition of boundaries is, "a line that marks the limits of an area; a dividing line." And as for personal boundaries, they are the limits and rules we set for ourselves within relationships. Whether it's with our friends, co-workers, family, and even strangers. When you are dealing with a traumatic experience, such as mine, you have to set boundaries in place so that you can properly heal, not just physically, but also mentally and spiritually.

For the most part of my life, I thought I had set pretty good and solid boundaries in place for myself and my family. But, I was being attacked in so many ways. I could not understand, for the life of me, why. My husband and I were pretty well-spoken when it came to telling friends and family what we stood for and what we did not. I truly wished I had the book of boundaries to give to some of my family and friends. What I experienced throughout my journey, no one could understand why or how I did things. One thing for sure, is it's not meant for anyone to understand when it's not their journey. However, that didn't stop anyone from saying or doing the things they did.

When I first told some of my family and friends I had been diagnosed with breast cancer, I only told a select few for my own peace. I requested that they respect my wishes of not telling anyone until I was ready. I am a firm believer in telling people what you want or don't want. If you don't, you will allow others to just run over you. Being that my family knows how private I am, at times, and don't allow a lot of people in my business, I assumed they would most definitely respect my wishes in this situation. However, that was not the case.

I had a relative pay me a visit shortly after I had recovered from my first chemo treatment. In all honesty, I was happy to see them. It was a great fellowship that lasted for hours. I shared with them my experience with taking chemotherapy. I cried, laughed, and talked with them about very personal things that were on my heart. I was so comfortable with them, even though it had been years since we last saw one another, but we had always kept in contact so it didn't matter.

Many of my family members did not know how badly my body rejected the treatment. All they knew was I had gotten sick, and I had come back to get my kids to take them back home. I didn't have to explain to anyone my decision. If I did give you that sacred info, that was my choice. When my relative left that evening I received a text that stated,

Good morning,
I know we haven't spoken in a while. I pray you're feeling better. Please don't close doors that have been open for you. You have to fight to live. Yes, your first treatment was harsh, but you can't give up now. You must think about what you had to endure when you were giving birth to your children. You did it without any medications and praise God you are blessed to have three beautiful children. Please continue your treatments. Don't ask how I know that you want to stop. No one told me. My spirit is connected with your spirit. DON'T GIVE IN TO CANCER YOU ARE A WINNER. I LOVE YOU!"

I immediately became angry! I screamed, threw things, and instantly called my husband. If anyone felt my pain I knew he would. I couldn't believe what I had just received. Here I was just getting through one of the scariest obstacles of my life. I was mad at the fact that I was violated in my own home by someone who I loved and trusted. Then for someone to tell me to continue to take the treatments and compare me having a natural birth to me experiencing death right before my eyes.

See, I never told anyone how I was knocking at death's door with only taking one chemo treatment. It is possible for a person to die from taking chemotherapy. However, many people do not talk about it, because they don't predict them dying from taking it. When I talked with my husband and told him what happened, he too became very upset. For one, he was upset with the person who came into our home and took advantage of me, at my most vulnerable state. We were brought up that what goes on in my house stays in my house, and you do not disclose personal information that was shared with you without permission. He was also very upset for the other relative to write me not even knowing what I had been through, and used God to talk me into not stopping my treatments.

We both called that person on three-way. It wasn't a very pleasant conversation. They tried to backtrack and wouldn't be honest with the information that was given and it pissed me off even more. They halfway apologized and said they would never call or text me again. That was short-lived as time went on. One day, I had had enough. I stopped picking up the phone and returning texts so that they could understand I have boundaries that will not be crossed. If you don't set solid boundaries, it will make you stressed out to the point that your physical body will break down and stress can kill you.

In the midst of all the attacks, I found an amazing Holistic Naturopathic doctor to assist me in my healing. I needed to heal my mind, body and spirit. On our first call, she prayed with me. She told me that I could not allow the burdens of my grandmother to have such a negative effect on me. I knew exactly what she meant, and it broke me down.

Over the years of me going through life's obstacles as a child, teenager and young adult, I always leaned on my grandmother to pray with me and for me. She had always been my go-to person when I needed someone to talk to about anything that troubled me. But, some secrets I kept to myself, because of guilt and shame. And, many of those secrets included her that I buried deep inside.

My grandmother was good at carrying everyone's issues and problems. She was a natural-born nurturer and healer. She had boundaries, but at times would bend them just to help that person, because of the title they held or not to have any conflicts with them altogether. She held so many things in and had nowhere to turn to for a release of her own. Her saying was she only needed to talk to God and her husband. But, many things throughout her life weighed heavy on her like anyone else may be experiencing.

I personally never had a therapist or talked with anyone outside of my circle. I was never taught about seeking professional help, only heard of those things through T.V. I knew I could not do it alone. For the next eight months, I worked hand and hand with Dr. Lisa to heal my mind, body and spirit while attacking this ugly disease aggressively from every angle possible.

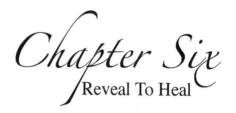

Chapter Six
Reveal To Heal

When we are faced with a shocking diagnosis, we may question ourselves or even God as to how or why this has happened. For me, once I got the information I had been diagnosed with breast cancer and evaluated the timing and everything that was surrounding the situation, I knew it was God's way of getting my attention. See, I have been through quite a bit for a twenty-nine-year-old; a victim of molestation as a young child, physical abuse, had a gun pulled on me as a young adult, and so many other traumatic experiences. And, one thing I've been able to do is to keep it suppressed and not allow it to overcome me. But, even that comes with its own set of problems. Because I did not deal with each situation, I became unhealthy physically and mentally.

Once I started my holistic treatments with Dr. Lisa, she pointed out to me various things that had come to her attention. Through scans she had done on me, she was able to help me understand my cancer, and what needed to be done to help. She pinpointed that I had been angry with someone. That was very much true. I was angry with God.

Yes, I was angry at God for taking my grandmother away, not allowing me to hear her voice before she departed, and for not healing her in a miraculous way. I was also angry at God for me having to deal with the same ugly disease that took my grandmother away. I was also angry at myself for allowing it to invade my body.

I was a person who always needed to be in control of my life. I didn't like surprises that I didn't know the answer to. Don't get me wrong. I love God and I know he loves me. However, at that present moment, I could not understand why I had to go through it without my grandmother being with me.

As I continued going to my appointments, more issues came about and one was forgiveness. That was alarming to me. I honestly felt that I didn't need to forgive anyone. I was perfectly fine with knowing what was done to me by people who did me wrong. I was content with not thinking or speaking of them ever again. In this case, I knew that in order for me to heal I would have to reveal things that I had once buried so deep that bringing it out was going to become very challenging. I was not ready, but understood it was necessary.

We began grief counseling. The first issue we brought up was of my grandmother. Why did I feel so angry towards God for allowing her to die suddenly? I cried like a baby during our first session. All I could say was she's supposed to be here with me and it isn't fair. See, my grandmother was my everything. She was a praying and strong woman; the person who I called on for everything. She would always be there. I knew she was in a much better place, where she didn't have to feel pain or sadness. But, it didn't make it any easier. She was gone. I had so much I wanted to ask her. So much I wanted to tell her. Being in my new home, in a new state, I felt alone and the only person who usually would fill that void was my grandma. Just a phone call would do.

It took weeks for me to finally have a breakthrough and allow myself to let go of the anger and embrace all the love and beautiful lessons my grandmother left me. I can say she left me with a strong will to love and serve God through all of life's battles. No matter what came to the surface, she reminded me whatever I did in my past or what happened to me in my past did not define me, and that God's purpose for my life was specifically for me. She would tell me that he is the only one who created me and knows what I can and cannot bear.

I was blessed to have such a wonderful woman who was selfless and dedicated her life to serving God and others through his word. Her journey on this earth was fulfilled. I had to let her go, but know that she is with me every step of my life. Man, that felt so beautiful and good to allow myself to let go of that burden and anger. It takes so much time and energy being mad at the world for something God has already ordained and there's nothing you can do about it. So, in that moment and going forth, I was done with being angry at God. I embraced his love and grace he has over my life.

Our next session was very unique. The type of therapy I attended was called RainDrop Therapy. It's a massage technique that uses various essential oils to help pull emotions from within and soothes inflammation and pain. The technique eases respiratory discomfort, enhances positive emotions, helps relieve stress, and supports the body to come back into balance. She wanted to use this technique to help me with forgiveness and the only way to reveal what needs to be forgiven is to talk about the issues that stop you from forgiving that person. For four hours, I allowed myself to relieve all the hurt and pain I endured that I blamed myself, my mother, my father, and the man who molested me for.

I experienced such a whirlwind of emotions that I had always felt deep down inside. I had suppressed them so well that I became numb to things and people, but I showed up smiling, even though I felt so broken inside. I had a great childhood, but the exposure I went through was a great deal that I wish I had never experienced, because of how painful it was.

My parents were young when they had me. They loved me dearly. But, with being raised by young parents, you are with them through many stages and challenges of their lives. Sometimes, the decisions they've made could have a negative or positive effect on you. Whether they understand it or not. My mother married young and the man she married seemed to be a great man for her. Many others did not agree.

He came into my life at a young age, as a toddler. I grew up calling him daddy and enjoyed having a dad in the house, even though he wasn't my biological dad. As I became older and aware, I saw the abuse my mother endured and I couldn't help her. Not too shortly after I became aware of the abuse, I too became a victim of his. I was beaten for stupid things that a child should not be punished for. I was even slapped in the face with a book, because I couldn't spell a word correctly at only six years old. I was so hurt and scared. The very man I called daddy abused me and my mother like it was nothing, and in the same breath said he loves me.

He started molesting me around the age of seven or eight. I was afraid to tell my mother, because of the abuse she was enduring as well. Honestly, I didn't know how she would respond, or what he would do to me if he found out I told. I did not see her ability to help me.

As the session continued, I experienced an outpour of hurt and a cry for help. I wanted to forgive every person who played a part in my life that I felt failed me at some point. I couldn't shake the fact that it was done to me and no one protected me. Even when I spoke up years later.

I understood and allowed myself to let go of a lot of the hurt and pain I had kept in for so long. I forgave myself for blaming myself for the things that were out of my control.

I also forgave my parents for exposing me to challenging times. But, I also thanked them for it. These times gave me a strength I never knew I had. I also understood they had their own traumas they may have been dealing with. Their traumas also played a part in a lot of their decisions throughout my childhood. I chose to love them through it all.

Dealing with cancer, you start to look and think about things from your past that you've never had the courage to deal with. God sits you down for you to deal with it so that you can heal properly. Those things of your past are not allowed to be a dark cloud over your life. I've always wanted to have a deep honest conversation with my parents, but never seem to have the courage to do so. Some of the times, when I have tried to talk it over with them it turns into a shouting match that never gets to the real truth.

Revealing my past and unveiling the truth of why I had been so angry, lifted a thousand pounds off of my shoulders. I was now ready to move forward with life without the feelings of anger and being unwanted. Dr. Lisa was such a blessing. However, I knew with just that one session I would still need continuous practice so that I wouldn't go back into that dark place.

I continued to go to my monthly appointments. I began

to gain the strength to learn as much as possible to heal my mind, body and spirit. I wasn't going to stop until I had a clean bill of health. With my husband by my side, it was much easier to do what needed to be done. I was ready for it.

Chapter Seven
Intimacy

Let's be honest with ourselves for a minute. When we dream to be married, what are some of the traits we want our significant other to have? Is it a man who is a leader, God-fearing, hard worker, compassionate and sexy? Personally, I asked God for a man who would be an amazing provider. Not just a provider financially, but one who will provide for himself and for his family like his life depended on it. I also asked God for my husband to be my best friend. One who I could talk to about any and everything, and enjoy all that life has to offer. I also asked God for a man who would protect me and love me unconditionally flaws and all.

Well, I prayed for my husband at the young age of twelve years old not knowing or understanding the power of the tongue. All I saw around me was how much my grandparents on both my mom's and dad's sides loved each other so much. I saw how both my grandfathers loved and cared for my grandmothers when they were battling cancer and how my grandmothers stood by my grandfather's side when they too went through their sickness over the years. My dad's mom, a survivor of breast cancer, was married to my grandfather for over fifty years before he passed. Seeing them together gave me so much joy and hope that I would have such a great man to love me the way my grandfather loved and cared for my grandmother. Then, there were my grandparents on my mom's side who I adored so much. They showed me the power of a praying couple and how through sickness and in death you are one.

On March 23, 2007, I met my husband whom I had prayed for. I did not know we would meet seven years later. We are high school sweethearts from the same side of the tracks. We went to the same school from pre-k all the way to high school, hung around the same friends, and we never knew or saw one another until my ninth-grade year in high school. I was actually dating someone at the time we met. I guess Mr. Kenneth was not having that and made his move. He took me from that young man. From that day on, I fell in love and we became such great friends from day one. As the years went on, we fell in and out as most young couples do. But, no matter where life took us, we always stayed connected.

One day, as I sat home, in a daze, I heard a voice say, "Kenneth Watts Jr. is your husband." As crazy as that may sound, I believed it. However, I wasn't too sure when it would happen or if it would really happen. I mean I was only eighteen years old and not ready to be anyone's wife so young; just enjoying being single and exploring the world. My thing was I wanted him to myself, but I wasn't ready to settle down just yet. And, I didn't think he was either.

He was pretty established at such a young age. What high schooler you know has his own mustang, great paying job, and isn't cocky with having such great things going for himself. Not to mention a few of the girls at school were after him and always wanted to fight me. Yes, he was something else, but mine.

As time passed, we went our separate ways. He graduated high school then joined the military. I graduated high school after him and left our hometown and pursued further schooling in Tallahassee, Florida. I ended up moving back to our hometown after a year. I was not too happy about being back.

Kenneth and I eventually reconnected and were in a long-distance relationship. With Kenneth across the country in Germany, I made the best of being home. But, I always knew I wanted more out of life, and to move out of my hometown and start a new life and career.

Kenneth would come home as much as he could, but would always have to leave out again. And again, that would always break my heart. In 2012, Kenneth got orders to be in Afghanistan. I was devastated. He had already been so far away for so long. Hearing that he had to go to such a dangerous place was a lot for me. So, I prayed daily for his safety. We talked as much as we could. It wasn't easy.

I eventually moved away to Atlanta, Georgia to pursue my acting and modeling career, which I had dreamed about for so long. Kenneth was happy for me as well.

I enjoyed everything about being in Atlanta, and the opportunities I was introduced to. All of the people I met were amazing. I was so happy to be there. Several months into staying with a family member, I was told I had to leave with no explanation. With nowhere to go or much money, I found myself sleeping from house to house and even in my car at times. This was something that I had never experienced and it was devastating.

When Kenneth gave me the news he was coming home and would be for good, I was more than ecstatic. I was ready to see him after two long years. I had found a townhome, but would not be able to move into it for several weeks. So, I decided to go home and pay Kenneth a visit which changed our lives forever. We have always had a special bond with being apart from one another and all that life had thrown our way. But, we seemed to hold onto each other this go around.

I ended up moving back to Pensacola and moving in with him. This was very scary. I had never stayed with any man. I didn't know what my grandparents would say about me shacking up. Even as an adult, I still cared for and respected their wishes. We then became pregnant with our firstborn son, Keiden. On August 16, 2014. I walked down the aisle to be married eight months pregnant. This was the best day of my life.

Three days later, after returning home from our honeymoon, my water broke and Keiden J. Watts was born. I thought life couldn't get any better, but God wasn't done. Through many challenges, throughout our marriage, God has a very unique way of showing both of us how he is with us; just as long as we are keeping him first and doing what it is that he has set forth for us.

Two years later, we were blessed with a beautiful baby girl. I had already named as a young girl picking names for me and Kenneth's future children in high school. God did exactly what I had prayed. We received our sweet princess, Serenity Rena Watts. At that moment, our little family was complete with a boy and a baby girl.

My life had become a fairytale. One that I was actually living. Marrying my high school sweetheart and having our own family was so amazing. It was such a blessing to be with someone who would be there with you through all of life's experiences; from being kids to now married with our own children. However, life can do a number on you that will test your marriage and it is not much you can do to prepare for it.

Now, here we are six years into our marriage with our third and last child, Zaccheaus, and in our new home in a new state. We moved to Atlanta following God's plan for our family which was for Kenneth to receive his doctorate degree in chiropractic. I would be expanding my wedding planning business, which I had been working on for four years. We loved our new home and starting a new life with our family. But, as the months went on, I found myself unable to enjoy our new life. I was battling the death of my grandmother and also postpartum had crept in and it had me down. Kenneth realized that something was not right, but didn't know exactly what it may have been. During this time he was such an amazing husband, surprising me with flowers just being a shoulder to lean on.

When we got the news of my breast cancer diagnosis, it was such a low blow for us. We were so young and had so much more life to achieve. The goals and plans we had set into place seemed challenging to obtain. I couldn't help but wonder if he would still look at me the same with me now having cancer in my body.

See, sex is not the only intimacy you need as a couple. You need someone to be there for you emotionally when you can't grasp life at times. Having to grieve the loss of a parent can take a toll on you. You need someone to care for you spiritually. At times, we are so caught up in the things we see happening with our physical eye and can't seem to find the strength to pray for ourselves. I thank God he blessed me with an amazing man to help me stay on track with God.

As the days, weeks, and months went on, life hit us in every way possible. I can honestly say it brought us even closer than ever before. With no family to lean on, during this challenging time, there was only us and our children. We were not prepared for what was ahead, but our love and strong will to stick by one another was all we needed.

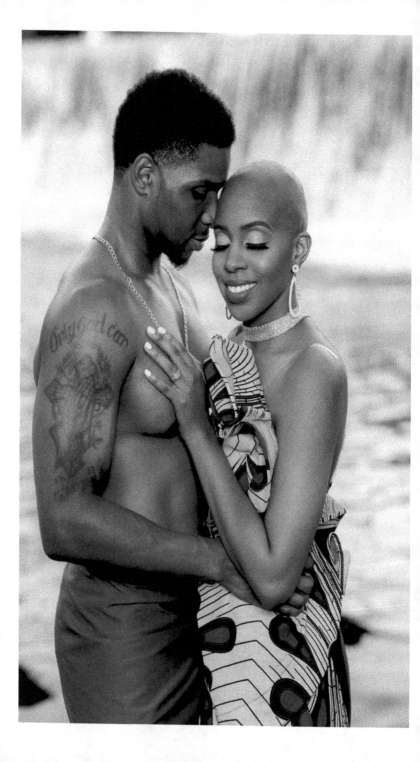

Chapter Eight
Uncomfortable

For eight months, I only ate a plant-based diet with fruits and spring water. I watched my tumor shrink right before my eyes. It was so astonishing to see the transformation. Just as I got comfortable with the amazing changes of my body and the healing that was taking place, I then started to see a change in my breasts and experienced excruciating pain all over my body. I talked with Dr. Lisa about what I was experiencing. My breasts had started to swell and I found small blister-like bumps forming upon my breast.

It was so detrimental to see what was happening right before my eyes. I was unsure what to do. I had been very strict on my diet, for the most part, and exercised as much as possible. To see what was happening caught me off guard. I prayed and prayed for God to not allow me to experience any pain or for my tumor to break through the skin. As time went on, it was something new happening every week. I found myself slipping back into that dark space where I would cry out to God to help me, but I didn't seem to get an answer.

It became very scary for me. I could not understand the attack that I was under physically, mentally and spiritually. Here I was balled up on my floor screaming to the top of my lungs, because of how bad my pain was. My husband is trying his best to console me, but was unable to be of any help. My children watched me drag myself across the floor. I was unable to walk or stand up straight, because my intestines were swollen from having C-diff (infection of the intestine).

At that time, I began to get down to the point I no longer had the desire to live. I no longer wanted to suffer or my family to see me in such a bad space. One night, all I could do was rock myself back and forth, because of the pain I was experiencing. I looked down at my breast and couldn't stand to look at how they were in such bad shape. Days had passed by with me being in intolerable pain and now my left arm had become ice cold and numb to the touch.

I decided to go to the emergency room as instructed by my doctor to be assured that I didn't have any blood clots or a blood infection. As I entered the hospital, I was told no one could accompany me due to the COVID-19 restrictions. I was upset that I could not have my husband or children with me in such a trying time. I was very nervous to go by myself. I desperately wanted my husband to be there with me, as he held my hand at that very moment. But, I had no choice, but to go in by myself to see what was happening to me.

After waiting patiently to see a doctor, I was finally seen after three hours. They ran tests on me and everything came back great; no blood infection or blood clots. My labs were so good that they were shocked that I had cancer. I explained to her that I had taken chemo once, but was unable to continue the treatments and was treating my cancer holistically. She immediately told me I was going to die in a few months. I could not believe what she was saying to me.

I became so enraged that she would say such a thing over me. Who was she to tell me I would die without any evidence of me dying. Only saying such a thing because I choose not to take chemo. I was already battling so many things in my head as to overcoming cancer. It wasn't easy going against the conventional way of treating cancer. However, I was not your average person to do things the way the world says you should do it.

As I stood there in front of the doctor, I went off like a firecracker, letting her know that I would not allow her or anyone else to speak death over my life. God is the one and the only person who has any say-so over my life, and death was not part of the plan. Being that I was not taking the conventional route for my healing, it did not sit well with many doctors I had seen during my many visits of trying to have the tumor removed or being able to have scans done to see my progress.

Life became very uncomfortable for myself and my

family. I would have to go by myself to various appointments and ER visits in the wee hours of the morning. Sometimes, I had to wake the children in the middle of the night to only be dropped off and sit in waiting rooms for hours and hours at a time. I didn't understand why God was allowing me to endure so much. However, I had to find the strength to hold onto God's promise he had made me at the beginning of my journey; "It Is Not Unto Death."

So, if it meant I had to be uncomfortable just a little while longer, I was willing to hold on just a little while longer. The pain over the next few weeks and months seemed to linger around with no remorse. I tried seeking help from other medical doctors as well as holistic doctors and nothing seemed to help.

My husband and I flew to Dallas, Texas to meet with a new doctor. By this time, Dr. Lisa had jumped ship. She was no longer responding to my calls or texts. I did not understand what was happening. All I could see was my body changing so drastically right in front of my eyes and it was scary to see.

Once we arrived in Dallas, my health took a turn for the worse. I was now unable to walk or sleep. It was driving me insane. The new doctor ran various tests on me and set me up with a new nutrition plan and many different supplements to take.

As we made it back home to start the new protocol, I couldn't help but think about how bad things had gotten since we had arrived back home in Atlanta. I hadn't slept in weeks, unable to lay flat in the bed or even close my eyes with so much pain all over my body.

Doctors would not do anything for me unless I agreed to take chemo and I was not having it. The pain was a part of me now for several months and prayer was not my first defense tool anymore. I had gotten so uncomfortable and constantly looked for an outlet for help to alleviate all the pain I was enduring. God had other plans, and I was unaware of what would happen next.

September 15, 2020

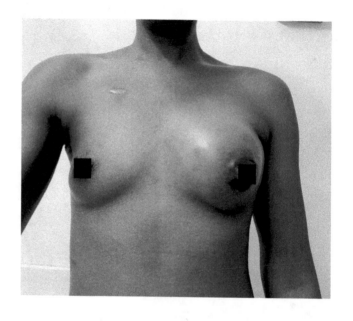

October 2, 2020

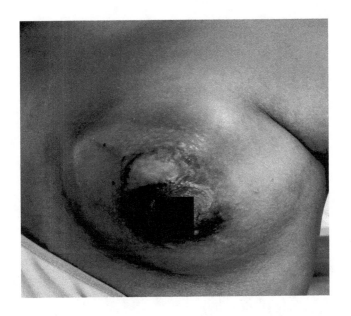

October 26, 2020

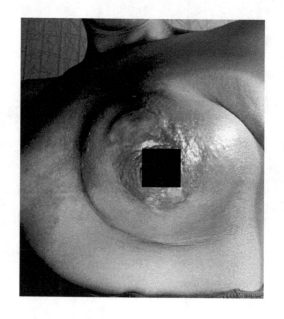

November 5, 2020

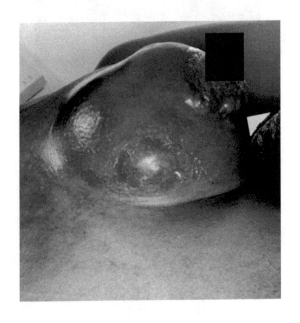

November 16, 2020

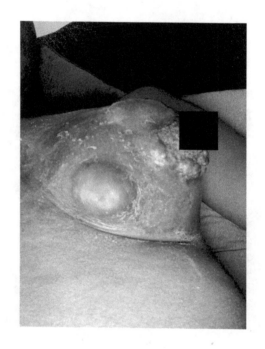

December 24, 2020

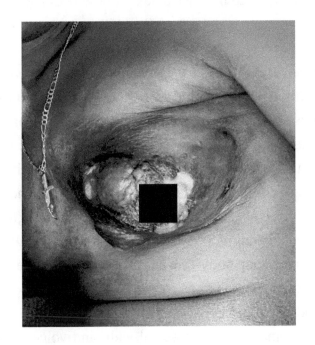

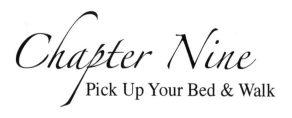

Chapter Nine
Pick Up Your Bed & Walk

Jesus saith unto him, Rise, take up thy bed, and walk.
~ John 5:8 (KJV)

For several weeks, I was unable to sleep or eat a full meal without experiencing some sort of pain. I started to lock myself away in my room, in the dark, just waiting for God to take me with him. It seemed like every time I would go into that dark space, my door would open with one of my babies or my husband coming in to check on me or just be in my presence. I was so weak and tired, unable to grasp what was happening to me. I had seen firsthand how cancer could break your body down, but it's nothing like experiencing it for yourself.

I had seen how my beautiful grandmother went from being a woman with a powerful walk and voice to unable to walk or talk. And, that's all I could think about was me going through what she had experienced. Was I wrong for thinking such things and not believing that God would bring me through this ugly disease? Would my children be left without a mother and my husband be left without a wife? I had so many questions for God and as I asked and cried out. I couldn't seem to get an answer back.

One particular Thursday afternoon, it was nothing too special, only that I had an urge to go for a walk. I called out to my husband to help me up so I could walk outside. As he held me up, I had to coach myself out loud, "Left, right, left, right. Kenisyha, you got this keep pushing." It took every ounce of me to keep walking.

We got outside and I continued to walk. As I pressed to walk, I heard a voice say, "RUN." I looked at my husband and said, "God says, Run!" I took off into a full sprint like never before. It was so shocking to feel my body with so much strength and power from just being unable to hold myself up.

Kenneth was right by my side to catch me, and I collapsed in his arms. He carried me back home. I went into a deep sleep for two hours. Something I had not been able to do for weeks. When I awakened, I walked into the living room and told my husband, "God said, 'Pick Up Your Bed and Walk. It's now time to go home for your healing.'" I knew exactly what he meant by going home to our home-town Pensacola, Florida. I didn't know what was awaiting us, but neither I nor my husband questioned God.

My husband packed all of our bags and made a few phone calls to our family in Florida. By 1:00 am, we were all packed in our truck and heading to Pensacola with no knowledge of what was about to take place or when we would return. We arrived in Pensacola on November 17, 2020. Our families welcomed us with open arms, others were a bit taken back by how bad my condition looked. I was barely able to walk and a whopping ninety-four pounds. It was mind bottling being back home with no direction as to which way to go.

After only being home for two days, I was rushed to the hospital. Several doctors and nurses in and out of my room constantly advising me I need to reconsider chemotherapy. I stayed in the hospital for a week and eventually was discharged on Thanksgiving Day.

The next day, I started experiencing trembles unaware that I was having a seizure. I told my husband to take me to a different hospital and thank God he did. Many tests and labs were taken to see what was causing me to have seizures. Once the results came back, it was revealed that I had a tumor on the right side of my brain. When I received the news, I couldn't believe what I was hearing, a tumor on my brain? How could this be? I had just gotten a scan back home in Atlanta and there was no indication that the cancer had spread anywhere in my body.

On December 10, 2020, I went under the knife to have brain surgery. Many prayers were in effect for me which calmed my spirit to not worry about the unknown. The surgery was a success and the nurses were so amazed at how well I was doing fresh out of surgery. They kept saying to me that I have a special guardian angel with me, because of how I was glowing during and after surgery. I could only respond back and say it's nobody but God who shines his light upon me.

God knew exactly what needed to be done and who needed to be in place during my time in the hospital. It's been eighteen long challenging months and that's only the tip of my journey which God has placed me upon. I still question God as to why I am having to go through such a trying time, but he always gives me signs that I am more than equipped to go through it all whether I know it or not.

I am still not cleared from being cancer-free. I had a long deep conversation with God about taking chemo again and he gave me the go. I truly believe the journey I had to endure was for a far better testimony to be given than God healing me from cancer from the start.

A few weeks later, after having brain surgery, I walked into my new oncologist's office and agreed to take chemo which would be six rounds. I prayed over it and went in trusting and believing God would allow the treatments to do what needed to be done and not take me under. He kept his promise, and I can thank Him for that. Now I am waiting for a total healing and a clean bill of health.

I've asked God every day when this will all be over and I have yet to receive an answer as to when. Nevertheless, no matter what life throws my way, I will continue to receive my "Healing By Faith".

So, what has happened now that I am done with chemo? Will I now be able to return back home? When will I have the tumor removed from my breasts? Just know God isn't done with this testimony quite yet. So, keep your seatbelt on as I continue to take you on this journey of faith.

Beautiful Struggle
The Journey

Releasing December 2022

ZYIA CONSULTING
Illuminate & Transcend

CPSIA information can be obtained
at www.ICGtesting.com
Printed in the USA
JSHW030438210622
27294JS00006B/182